An Analysis of Marijuana Policy

Committee on Substance Abuse and Habitual Behavior
Commission on Behavioral and Social Sciences and Education
National Research Council

National Academy Press
Washington, D.C. 1982

NOTICE: The project that is the subject of this report was approved by the Governing Board of the National Research Council, whose members are drawn from the councils of the National Academy of Sciences, the National Academy of Engineering, and the Institute of Medicine. The members of the committee responsible for the report were chosen for their special competences and with regard for appropriate balance.

This report has been reviewed by a group other than the authors according to procedures approved by a Report Review Committee consisting of members of the National Academy of Sciences, the National Academy of Engineering, and the Institute of Medicine.

The National Research Council was established by the National Academy of Sciences in 1916 to associate the broad community of science and technology with the Academy's purposes of furthering knowledge and of advising the federal government. The Council operates in accordance with general policies determined by the Academy under the authority of its congressional charter of 1863, which establishes the Academy as a private, non-profit, self-governing membership corporation. The Council has become the principal operating agency of both the National Academy of Sciences and the National Academy of Engineering in the conduct of their services to the government, the public, and the scientific and engineering communities. It is administered jointly by both Academies and the Institute of Medicine. The National Academy of Engineering and the Institute of Medicine were established in 1964 and 1970, respectively, under the charter of the National Academy of Sciences.

Available from:
Commission on Behavioral and Social Sciences and Education
National Research Council
2101 Constitution Avenue, N.W.
Washington, D.C. 20418
Printed in the United States of America

NATIONAL RESEARCH COUNCIL
2101 CONSTITUTION AVENUE WASHINGTON, D.C. 20218

OFFICE OF THE CHAIRMAN
June 21, 1982

Dr. William Pollin,
Director
National Institute on Drug Abuse Parklawn Building Room 10-05 5600 Fishers Lane Rockville, Maryland20857

Dear Dr. Pollin:

I transmit, herewith, a report of the National Research Council's Committee on Substance Abuse and Habitual Behavior: "An Analysis of Marijuana Policy" prepared at the request of the National Institute on Drug Abuse.

The Committee on Substance Abuse and Habitual Behavior, composed of 18 experts in the several relevant disciplines, has weighed carefully the available data regarding the costs, risks, and benefits of the major policy alternatives regarding the control of marijuana use and supply. The Committee is clear in pointing to the deficiencies of this body of evidence and cautions about the hazards of formulating policy recommendations based solely or in part thereon. In this regard, I call your attention to the following statement by Louis Lasagna and Gardner Lindzey contained in the Preface to the report:

> The Committee wishes to make clear what it regards as the limits of this report for the selection of policy alternatives. Scientific judgment can estimate the prevalence of different kinds of use, risks to health, economic costs, and the like under current policies and try to project such estimates for new policies. It can come to some conclusions based on those estimates. But selection of an alternative is always a value-governed choice, which can ultimately be made only by the political process.

This caveat notwithstanding, the Committee has derived from its examination of the scientific data a conclusion about the major policy choices facing the nation with respect to

THE NATIONAL RESEARCH COUNCIL IS THE PRINCIPAL OPERATING AGENCY OF THE NATIONAL ACADEMY OF SCIENCES AND THE NATIONAL ACADEMY OF ENGINEERING TO SERVE GOVERNMENT AND OTHER ORGANIZATIONS.

marijuana: complete prohibition, prohibition of supply only, and regulatory approaches. Specifically, the Committee concurs with the judgment of the National Commission on Marijuana and Drug Abuse, rendered in 1971, that a policy of prohibition of supply only is preferable to a policy of complete prohibition of supply and use.

What must be understood by the public, the media, and all who read the Committee's report is that its decision to endorse a policy change was not fashioned from scientific information--old or new--alone. Rather it was the analysis of a combination of factors which affect policy decisions, including the cost and efficacy of enforcement practices. Values were necessarily involved in balancing these factors and there are those within the membership and governing bodies of the Academies and the National Research Council who might not have come to the same policy conclusions, after reviewing the same data.

My own view is that the data available to the Committee were insufficient to justify on scientific or analytical grounds changes in current policies dealing with the use of marijuana. In this respect I am concerned that the Committee may have gone beyond its charge in stating a judgment so value-laden, that it should have been left to the political process.

I have one further concern that cannot go unaddressed. I fear that this report, coming as it does from a well-known and well-respected scientific organization, will be misunderstood by the media and the public to imply that new scientific data are suddenly available that justify changes in public attitudes on the use of marijuana. This would be unfortunate at a time when daily use trends by high school students are down significantly. As the Committee's discussion of marijuana's behavioral and health-related effects clearly demonstrates, there is no new scientific information exonerating marijuana. In fact, the review by our Institute of Medicine, published a few months ago, reevaluated existing scientific evidence and concluded, as have others, that marijuana is a harmful drug whose use justifies serious national concern.

I wish to remind you that this is a committee report; the only position that can be inferred with respect to the National Research Council on the issue of marijuana policy is that the National Research Council is satisfied that the Committee was competent to examine the issue and diligent in carrying out its task. Despite my personal disagreement, I believe that the Committee has performed a useful service by illuminating many of the complex issues surrounding this highly controversial subject.

Yours sincerely,

Frank Press
Chairman

COMMITTEE ON SUBSTANCE ABUSE AND HABITUAL BEHAVIOR

LOUIS LASAGNA (Chair), Department of Pharmacology and Toxicology, University of Rochester School of Medicine and Dentistry
HOWARD S. BECKER, Department of Sociology, Northwestern University
PETER DEWS, Department of Psychiatry and Psychobiology, Harvard University
JOHN L. FALK, Department of Psychology, Rutgers University
DANIEL X. FREEDMAN, Department of Psychiatry, University of Chicago
JEROME H. JAFFE, Veterans Administration Hospital, Newington, Connecticut, and University of Connecticut School of Medicine, Farmington, Connecticut
DENISE KANDEL, Department of Psychiatry and School of Public Health, Columbia University, and New York State Psychiatric Institute
JOHN KAPLAN, Stanford University School of Law
GARDNER LINDZEY (past chair), Center for Advanced Study in the Behavioral Sciences, Stanford, California
GERALD McCLEARN, College of Human Development, Pennsylvania State University
CHARLES P. O'BRIEN, Veterans Administration Hospital, Philadelphia, and Department of Psychiatry, University of Pennsylvania
JUDITH RODIN, Department of Psychology, Yale University
STANLEY SCHACHTER, Department of Psychology, Columbia University
THOMAS C. SCHELLING, John F. Kennedy School of Government, Harvard University
RICHARD L. SOLOMON, Department of Psychology, University of Pennsylvania

FRANK STANTON, New York (formerly, president, Columbia Broadcasting System)
ALBERT STUNKARD, Department of Psychiatry, University of Pennsylvania
RICHARD F. THOMPSON, Department of Psychology, Stanford University
PETER K. LEVISON, Study Director
DEAN R. GERSTEIN, Senior Research Associate
DEBORAH R. MALOFF, Research Associate
MARIE A. CLARK, Administrative Secretary

CONTENTS

PREFACE	xi
INTRODUCTION	1
THE DANGERS OF MARIJUANA	3
OVERVIEW OF CURRENT MARIJUANA POLICIES	6
A REVIEW OF THE REPORT OF THE NATIONAL COMMISSION ON MARIJUANA AND DRUG ABUSE	9
THE USE OF MARIJUANA: COMPARING COMPLETE AND PARTIAL PROHIBITION	11
Effects of Partial Prohibition	12
Costs of Prohibition of Use	14
Public Attitudes Toward Partial Prohibition	16
THE SUPPLY OF MARIJUANA: COMPARING PROHIBITED AND REGULATED MARKETS	17
Costs of Prohibition of Supply	18
Costs of Regulating Supply	20
Regulatory Systems: Some Concrete Aspects	24
CONCLUSIONS	29
RECOMMENDATIONS FOR RESEARCH	30
Health and Behavior	30
Drug Markets	31
Effects on Use	31
REFERENCES	33
APPENDIX: SUMMARY OF MARIJUANA AND HEALTH	36

PREFACE

In 1978 the Committee on Substance Abuse and Habitual Behavior began a study of marijuana policy at the request and with the support of the National Institute on Drug Abuse. Sharp increases in marijuana use along with suggestions for reform of existing marijuana laws from scientists and policy makers prompted a renewed look at those laws. In addition, the National Commission on Marijuana and Drug Abuse, in its 1973 final report, <u>Drug Use in America: Problem in Perspective,</u> had recommended that a follow-up commission be appointed to review possible changes in the situation four years later. That recommendation was not implemented, so the Committee took as a framework for its task the assessment that the Commission recommended, especially the assessment of new evidence regarding the effects of recent changes in state marijuana policies.

The Committee conducted its study with awareness of the intensity of past controversies about marijuana use in U.S. society. In the four years since the Committee began its work, there has been an increase in visible concern among many parents about marijuana use among youth, its potential risks to the health of children, and the possibility that heavy use by some young people may seriously threaten their education. Parents who have experienced problems with their own children, or observed those of others, have organized to make marijuana policies a major item on current political agendas. In comparison with the situation at the inception of this study, there is today greater rancor in public discussion, press reports, legislative hearings, and policy-oriented technical meetings related to marijuana use.

This is the context in which the Committee completed its review of the evidence and arguments of earlier studies and weighed the significance of subsequent evidence for the major policy alternatives. Every policy has potentially good and potentially bad effects, and policy choices involve difficult comparisons of such effects. It is important to recognize that to allow the inertia developed by existing policies to prevent change is itself a choice.

The Committee is aware that analyzing a topic that is the subject of heated social debate has its hazards. Many of those participating in the marijuana debate have already selected what they take to be the admissible terms of the discussion and look with disfavor on anyone's insistence on a wider set of considerations. For example, some would settle the issue on physiological grounds alone: whether cannabis products, in the dose ranges customarily used by most people, cause tissue damage. Defenders of marijuana use may seize on the ambiguity or absence of evidence for such damage and ignore any other effects on education or safety; those opposed to marijuana use may emphasize the possibility of chronic disease that is suggested by some laboratory findings and ignore the social, political, and economic costs of fighting a well-established custom.

This report does not review and analyze every conceivable policy nuance or option. It addresses the major choices--both because these families of alternative policies subsume many variants and because the choice among these major options must be discussed before specific, perhaps new, policy instruments can be designed.

The Committee wishes to make clear what it regards as the limits of this report for the selection of policy alteratives. Scientific judgment can estimate the prevalence of different kinds of use, risks to health, economic costs, and the like under current policies and can try to project such estimates for new policies. It can come to some conclusions based on those estimates. But selection of an alternative is always a value-governed choice, which can ultimately be made only by the political process. The role of scientific evidence in this process is not inconsiderable, even though, at times, the strongest evidence may be pushed aside and the wildest speculation prevail. But the weight of the evidence is only one factor in the process of policy formation; ultimately, that process involves value choices.

In completing its report, the Committee has benefited from many people in formulating, revising, and updating the analyses and data. A very early version of this report was discussed at the Committee's annual conference in 1979, and subsequent versions benefited from comments by staff of the National Institute on Drug Abuse and of the National Research Council. The final draft received close and constructive attention by members of the National Research Council's Commission on Behavioral and Social Sciences and Education, the Institute of Medicine, and the Report Review Committee of the National Academy of Sciences.

We have also maintained a close liaison with the staff and members of the Institute of Medicine's Committee to Study the Health-Related Effects of Cannabis and Its Derivatives, on which three members of our Committee also served, and whose recently published report, <u>Marijuana and Health,</u> significantly contributed to our work.

Two former Committee members, Troy Duster and Michael Agar, assisted in the early preparation of the report. At later stages we were very ably assisted by the staff of the Commission on Behavioral and Social Sciences and Education, in particular David Goslin, executive director, and Eugenia Grohman, associate director for reports. Without their help, it is doubtful that we could have completed this task. Finally, we are indebted to the staff and members of the Committee, for their diligence, patience, and commitment to a difficult assignment.

Louis Lasagna, Chair
Gardner Lindzey, Chair, 1977-1980
Committee on Substance Abuse and Habitual Behavior

An Analysis of Marijuana Policy

INTRODUCTION

Since the early 1960s the use of marijuana as an intoxicant by a growing proportion of the American population has been an issue of major national concern. Despite repeated warnings of possible adverse health consequences and persistent efforts by law enforcement agencies to restrict the supply and use of marijuana, available data indicate that experimentation with or regular use of the drug is no longer restricted to a small minority of Americans. In 1979, for example, 68 percent of young adults between the ages of 18 and 25 reported having tried marijuana; 35.4 percent reported having used marijuana in the last month. Among adults over age 26, the proportion having ever used marijuana has more than doubled since 1971, from 9.2 percent to 19.6 percent (Fishburne et al., 1980; see Table 1, below).

Although "the marijuana problem" may be viewed as of recent origin, marijuana is not a new drug. The cannabis plant has been cultivated and used both for its intoxicating properties and for its fiber (hemp) throughout the world for more than 10,000 years (Abel, 1980). At various times and places attempts have been made to restrict its use as an intoxicant; at other times and places its virtues have been extolled for medical purposes, and it has played a significant role in religious ritual. Because cannabis is easily grown--indeed, it is one of the hardiest of all plant species--its resin has been used for centuries along with tobacco, fermented distillates of grains and fruits (alcohol), and opium derivatives as one means of relieving stresses associated with daily life.

INTRODUCTION

Despite its long history, the use of cannabis as an intoxicant was relatively unknown in the United States until the latter part of the nineteenth century, and even then its use as a drug was restricted to a tiny fraction of the population, primarily immigrants from Mexico. The first efforts to restrict its use in this country did not occur until 1911, when Congress, which at that time was considering proposals for federal antinarcotics legislation, listened to arguments that cannabis should be included in the list of illegal drugs. That effort failed, but during the next two decades a number of state legislatures moved to prohibit the possession of marijuana unless prescribed by a physician. It was not until 1937, when the Marijuana Tax Law was enacted, that the federal government became involved in the attempt to control its use. Even this law recognized the industrial uses of hemp and also exempted the seeds of the plant, which were then being sold as bird feed. In 1956, Congress included marijuana in the Narcotics Act of that year and, in 1961, the United Nations adopted the Single Convention on Narcotic Drugs, the terms of which state that each participating country could "adopt such measures as may be necessary to prevent misuse of, and illicit traffic in, the leaves of the cannabis plant." Congress approved participation in the convention in 1967 and three years later passed the Comprehensive Drug Abuse Prevention and Control Act, which provides the basis for current federal prohibitions regarding marijuana use.

Despite this history it was not until the 1960s that most Americans became aware of marijuana. The political and cultural protests of that period focused public attention on young people, their life-styles, and their use of drugs, including marijuana. That period created the context in which public policies regarding marijuana use have been debated since the early 1970s. As Abel (1980) points out, for the first time marijuana use was not restricted to minority groups and fringe elements of society: many of the new users were native-born, middleclass, white college students. Without doubt, the political and cultural context in which marijuana emerged as an issue of national concern has strongly influenced the subsequent policy debate about its use.

The policy debate about marijuana use has also brought into sharp focus two conflicting but deeply held beliefs of large and overlapping segments of the American population. To many, the use of drugs of any kind solely for the purpose of producing states of intoxication is abhorrent, entirely apart from any presumed health effects. At the same time, many people strongly defend the right of individuals to privately indulge their desires, so long as others are not adversely affected. Adding to the complexity of the issues are continuing uncertainties about the health and developmental consequences of marijuana use, concern over the growing number of adolescent users, the social consequences of prosecuting otherwise law-abiding citizens for possession and use of marijuana, the relationship between the distribution of marijuana and that of other illegal drugs, the costs of enforcement of current laws, and the economic implications of the persistence of very large illegal markets.

The next section of this report presents a brief summary of existing evidence regarding the health consequences of marijuana use, drawing heavily on the recently completed study by the Institute of Medicine. The third section summarizes existing federal and state laws relating to the supply and use of marijuana. The fourth section of the report reviews the conclusions of the report of the National Commission on Marijuana and Drug Abuse (1972). The next two sections deal, respectively, with policies regarding the use and the supply of marijuana. The two final sections present a summary of the committee's conclusions regarding major policy options and recommendations for research needed to more adequately assess those options.

THE DANGERS OF MARIJUANA

Marijuana is not a harmless drug. Although available evidence suggests that marijuana may be less likely than opiates, barbiturates, or alcohol to induce psychological and physical dependence in its users, it has the capacity to reduce the effective functioning of individuals under its influence, and prolonged or excessive use may cause serious harmful biological and social effects in many users.

The recent report, Marijuana and Health, of the Institute of Medicine (1982:5 [reproduced in the appendix]) concludes:

> The scientific evidence published to date indicates that marijuana has a broad range of psychological and biological effects, some of

which, at least under certain conditions, are harmful to human health. Unfortunately, the available information does not tell us how serious this risk may be.

Overall, the report concludes (p. 5):

[W]hat little we know for certain about the effects of marijuana on human health--and all that we have reason to suspect--justifies serious national concern.

The complete summary of the Institute of Medicine report appears as the appendix to this report.

Over the past 40 years, marijuana has been accused of causing an array of antisocial effects, including: in the 1930s, provoking crime and violence; in the early 1950s, leading to heroin addiction; and in the late 1960s, making people passive, lowering motivation and productivity, and destroying the American work ethic in young people. Although beliefs in these effects persist among many people, they have not been substantiated by scientific evidence.

Concerns about how marijuana affects citizenship, motivation, and job performance have become less salient in recent years as marijuana has moved more into the mainstream of society and has become less exclusively associated with radicals, hippies, or disadvantaged minorities. Though there is still widespread belief that heavy marijuana use may be incompatible with a responsible, productive life, evidence that marijuana has not adversely affected either the productivity or the sense of social responsibility of some groups of users (see, e.g., Hochman and Brill, 1973) has tempered earlier fears of a widespread "amotivational syndrome." Research that correlates marijuana use with undesirable behavior, such as alienation or inattention to school studies, has not established the direction of causality or ruled out spurious associations (see, e.g., Beachy et al., 1979). This issue, however, continues to be the subject of lively controversy and the Institute of Medicine report (1982:125) concludes that "it appears likely that both self-selection and authentic drug effects contribute to the 'motivational' problems seen in some chronic marijuana users."

Recently, a body of literature has accumulated that reports on links between marijuana use and such health impairments as lung disease, chromosome damage, reduced reproductive function, and brain dysfunction (summarized in Institute of Medicine, 1982, and National Institute on Drug Abuse, 1980). In some areas--for example, effects on the nervous system and behavior and on the cardiovascular and respiratory systems--there is clear evidence that marijuana produces acute short-term effects (Institute of Medicine, 1982:2,3):

> With a severity directly related to dose, marijuana impairs motor coordination and affects tracking ability and sensory and perceptual functions important for safe driving and the operation of other machines. . . . [It also] increases the work of the heart, usually by raising the heart rate and, in some persons, by raising blood pressure.

There is as yet no such clear evidence on the possible long-term effects in these areas, or of other potential health consequences of marijuana use; further research is needed. In addition, most studies on human populations have been laboratory studies of young, healthy adult males. Differential effects of marijuana use on the elderly, on pregnant women, on groups that are psychiatrically vulnerable or at risk for disease or dysfunction, and particularly on adolescents have not been studied systematically.

In our view, the most troublesome aspects of marijuana use are its potential effects on the development of adolescents. Parents as well as a number of clinicians and researchers are concerned that the social and intellectual development of teenagers may be harmed by chronic marijuana use. There is good evidence that intoxication may seriously impair such important skills as comprehension and retention of newly presented educational materials (Institute of Medicine, 1982). Rapidly growing tissues have been shown to be particularly vulnerable to some, although by no means all, toxic agents, and there is at least a possibility that toxic effects may be subtle and not clearly manifest until adulthood. Scientifically, these are difficult relationships to identify, and the research to date is still insufficient to strongly support any relationship.

Perhaps more significant than any lasting biological effect is the effect of the drug in different patterns of use on emotional development, on the formation of habits, and on the acquisition of coping skills for stress situations. Indeed, although the many issues raised by the use of intoxicants to escape stressful challenge have not been systematically studied, the evident attractiveness of marijuana to many adolescents, and its possible dose-related interference with the study and hard work needed for intellectual development in the crucial high school years, make this a special matter for concern. This is particularly so in light of the fact that, unlike alcohol, marijuana is used by many adolescents during school hours. Finally, reports of the effects of marijuana use on automobile driving skills are worrisome.

This Committee has reviewed the scientific literature surveys of marijuana effects on health and behavior, including the major recent study conducted by the Institute of Medicine (1982) and those by the National Institute on Drug Abuse (1979; 1980), Tashkin et al. (1978), Nahas (1977), and Fried (1977). We agree with the conclusion of the Institute of Medicine report that it is likely that long-term heavy marijuana use will be shown to result in measurable damage to health, just as long-term chronic tobacco and alcohol use have proven to cause such damage. It is evident that the full impact of marijuana use on human health will not be clear without careful epidemiological studies involving substantial populations of users--a matter of some decades--even though it is predictable that this drug--like all others--will cause harm in some of its users, particularly in its heaviest users, and among these, in its heaviest adolescent users. At this time, however, our judgment as to behavioral and health-related hazards is that the research has not established a danger both large and grave enough to override all other factors affecting a policy decision.

OVERVIEW OF CURRENT MARIJUANA POLICIES

Current federal and state marijuana laws are in part governed by international treaty. The major federal law relevant to marijuana is the Comprehensive Drug Abuse Prevention and Control Act of 1970, which repealed all prior federal legislation and reduced federal penalties for possession and sale. Although marijuana possession and sale are still prohibited, possession has been reduced from a felony to a misdemeanor offense; the maximum penalty for a first offense is $5,000 and one year's imprisonment. The Act also provides for conditional dis-charge, by which first offenders found guilty of simple possession or casual transfer (which is treated as simple possession) may be placed on probation for up to one year (Congressional Digest, 1979).

The Uniform Controlled Substance Act of 1970, drafted by the National Conference of Commissioners on Uniform State Laws, was designed to make state laws more compatible with the new federal law. Like the federal act, the Uniform Act reclassified marijuana as a hallucinogen rather than a narcotic and reduced the penalty for possession from the felony to the misdemeanor level; a majority of the states have adopted the Uniform Act. Eleven states have withdrawn the criminal sanction from possession for personal use. In these states, arrest has been replaced with a traffic-ticket type of citation, and a small fine is the sole allowable penalty. About 30 states include some provision for conditional discharge of first offenders, and about a dozen of them provide for all records of the offense to be expunged. The Alaska Supreme Court ruled in 1975 that possession for personal use by adults at home was protected by the constitutional right to privacy and hence was not subject to any penalty (Rosenthal, 1979).

State penalties for second-offense possession and for selling marijuana are extremely variable. (See National Organization for the Reform of Marijuana Laws and Center for Study of Non-Medical Drug Use, 1979, for summary tables of state marijuana laws.) Sale is almost always a felony, with maximum sentences ranging from two years to life, although casual transfer, or "accommodation," is sometimes exempt from felony treatment. All but 15 jurisdictions punish cultivation as heavily as they do sale; the Uniform Act includes the two in the same classification (manufacture), with the same penalty provisions.

Federal prohibition of small-scale possession is virtually unenforced. At the March 1977 House of Representatives hearings on decriminalization, the chief of the criminal division of the Department of Justice testified that the federal government no longer effectively prosecutes the use of marijuana, "nor do we, under any conceivable way, in the Federal Government have the resources to do so" (Select Committee on Narcotics Abuse and Control, 1977:13). In terms of its effects from a law enforcement point of view, the present official federal policy of complete prohibition does not differ in fact from a policy of prohibition of supply only. Complete prohibition is the federal law, but partial prohibition is the practice. However, the law, even though partly unenforced, has probably had a restraining influence on the willingness of states to adopt policies of less than complete prohibition. The states traditionally have followed the federal lead in drug abuse legislation, although they are not legally required to do so (see the testimony of Jay Miller, American Civil Liberties Union, to the Select Committee on Narcotics Abuse and Control, 1977). In summary, in most states and according to federal law, U.S. marijuana policy is one of complete prohibition--that is, prohibition of both supply and use.

Major alternatives to complete prohibition include prohibition of supply only--called partial prohibition--and regulation.* Prohibition of supply only means having no penalty (or only civil penalties) for use, possession, or, sometimes, "casual transfer" of small quantities of marijuana, while having criminal penalties for manufacture, importation, or commercial sale of marijuana. Regulation means not only eliminating penalties for use but also allowing controlled production and distribution.

Within each of the three broad policy options--complete prohibition, prohibition of supply only, and regulation--numerous subsidiary policy choices exist. For example, a policy of complete prohibition necessitates decisions about the resources to be devoted to enforcement, the appropriate penalties to be imposed for violations, and whether marijuana should be made available for any medical uses. Under a policy of prohibition of supply only, decisions must still be made about penalties and permitted medical uses. In addition, one must also determine how to distinguish between users

---

*In this discussion, we use the terms "complete prohibition," and "prohibition of supply and use" interchangeably. We also use the terms "partial prohibition," "prohibition of supply only," and "decriminalization" as equivalent. We generally prefer the terms "partial prohibition," or "prohibition of supply only" since many people seem to regard decriminalization as the equivalent of legalization or regulation--which it most certainly is not. (The policy of partial prohibition has also been called the vice model.) Finally, we use "regulation" and "legalization" as equivalent terms.

and suppliers; whether cultivation should be permitted; how stronger preparations of the cannabis plant, such as hashish, should be treated; whether to criminalize small-scale casual transfers, made with or without payment; and what should be done about certain specific behaviors, such as the public use of marijuana and the operation of motor vehicles under the influence of the drug. Under a policy of regulation, some of the issues to be decided are the type of control system (e.g., state monopoly or licensed sale), the rules as to potency and quality, and appropriate penalties for violation of the system's rules.

The variety of choices within each of the broad policy options suggests that none can be characterized in a monolithic way. Some regulatory systems could be so stringent as to have results similar to prohibitory laws: e.g., a regulatory system that raised the price drastically above what the illegal market charges. Similarly, lack of enforcement could strongly reduce the impact of a prohibitory option. As we have already noted, this latter effect has already occurred in some jurisdictions in which the law provides for complete prohibition but users are not in fact prosecuted.

A REVIEW OF THE REPORT OF THE NATIONAL COMMISSION ON MARIJUANA AND DRUG ABUSE

An attempt to describe a full array of policy options together with associated benefits and detriments of each of them was made by the National Commission on Marijuana and Drug Abuse in its 1972 report, <u>Marijuana: A Signal of Misunderstanding</u>. With respect to the major policy choices, the Commission did a thorough job. The members and staff recognized the limited knowledge base for their deliberations and subsequently recommended that a second commission be appointed to review the situation four years later. Such a follow-up commission was never appointed. It seems appropriate, then, that this Committee reappraise the Commission's work in light of subsequent research findings, especially those relating to recent changes in marijuana policies.

The Commission examined the spectrum of social policies available to control marijuana use and the benefits and detriments of implementing each policy. The legal alternatives presented included those identified above: complete prohibition; prohibition of supply only; and regulatory approaches. The Commission emphasized that choosing among the three approaches requires consideration of the social milieu, cultural values, and practicalities of implementation. The Commission considered such social conditions particularly important in examining marijuana controls because both use of the drug and the laws prohibiting supply and use had symbolic importance, representing a clash of values between a dominant culture that opposed marijuana use and a large minority that either used marijuana or condoned its use. The probable effects of the various policies considered by the Commission include changes in use patterns, enforcement costs, and influence on related social concerns such as the marketing of other illicit drugs and general respect for law.

The Commission commented on all three broad policy options. It suggested first that total prohibition has resulted in costly enforcement, alienation of the young, discrimination through selective enforcement, some deterrence of supply (especially to middle-aged and middleclass potential users), but minimal deterrence of use by those with access to the drug. Second, the Commission stated its belief that prohibition of supply only would support the official policy of discouraging use, but at the same time would recognize the practical difficulties of attempting to eliminate use. The report listed a number of choices that might be made under a system of partial prohibition and described some of the practical problems they might entail (e.g., the need to distinguish between casual and commercial distributors). Finally, the Commission described regulation as a policy that only mildly disapproved of occasional use and that concentrated on controlling excessive use, but was mostly designed to lower the costs of prohibiting the drug. The Commission argued that marijuana consumption would increase considerably if complete prohibition were replaced by regulation. In addition, the Commission considered a major drawback of any regulatory system to be that its elimination of the main symbol of society's disapproval--criminal sanctions--would cause resentment among the nonuser majority of the population. Marijuana was described as being symbolic of countercultural lifestyles: "the drug's symbolism creates a risk of strong political reaction to any liberalization of the present laws by older members of the society" (National Commission on Marijuana and Drug Abuse, 1972, Appendix Volume II:1149).

On balance, the Commission concluded that, since the threat of punishment had not apparently deterred the millions of people who had already used marijuana, the replacement of complete by partial prohibition would not produce a significant increase in marijuana use. Consequently, the Commission recommended that individual marijuana users should not be subject to criminal prosecution for their private use or possession of small amounts of the drug, and that, on balance, the best policy was one of prohibition of supply only. In accordance with this view, the Commission recommended that federal and state laws should be amended to achieve partial prohibition. In the decade since the Commission report, a number of states have changed their laws in varying ways. These legal changes can be viewed as natural experiments, and one can use the data from them to reassess the Commission's conclusions regarding these policies.

THE USE OF MARIJUANA: COMPARING COMPLETE AND PARTIAL PROHIBITION

To compare the two types of marijuana control policies presently used in the United States--prohibition of supply and use and prohibition of supply only--we need to consider only the one particular in which they differ: the application of criminal sanctions against marijuana users. To compare the effects of the two policies, we can examine the effects of the prohibition of use and determine whether prohibition results in more costs than benefits or vice versa.

In recent years the prohibition of marijuana use has come under increasing criticism. Many students of the U.S. marijuana situation, including the National Commission on Marijuana and Drug Abuse, members of Congress, political analysts, and legal experts, have suggested that existing laws prohibiting marijuana use be repealed. These suggestions have been prompted by the failure of current policies to deter large numbers of users, the consequent criminalization of large numbers of young Americans, and the high social costs of such law enforcement. A number of professional associations and agencies have also gone on record in support of the removal of all criminal penalties for the private possession and use of marijuana as a means of reducing the economic costs of law enforcement and the social costs of arrest or imprisonment (criminalization) of young people who are otherwise not criminally involved or labeled. The organizations and agencies that have expressed this view include the American Medical Association, the American Bar Association, the American Public Health Association, the Canadian Commission of Inquiry into the Non-Medical Use of Drugs, the National Council of Churches, the National Advisory Commission on Criminal Justice Standards and Goals, the National Commission on Marijuana and Drug Abuse, among others. Eleven states, with one-third of the nation's population, have adopted some version of partial prohibition or "decriminalization." (In Oregon, Alaska, Maine, Colorado, California, Ohio, Minnesota, Mississippi, New York, North Carolina, and Nebraska, citations and small fines have replaced arrests and incarceration for use-only marijuana-related offenses.)

At first glance, criminalizing the selling of marijuana might appear inconsistent with failing to punish its purchase. But in the drafting of laws, a line is often drawn between legal and illegal conduct so that the maximum reduction in the proscribed behavior can be gained at minimum social cost. Frequently it turns out that laws aimed solely at suppressing sales are more cost-effective in reducing both the possession and use of a substance than are laws that attempt to suppress possession directly. There are several reasons for this. First, there are fewer sellers than buyers; this permits a concentration of law enforcement efforts where they do the most good. Second, juries are likely to be more sympathetic to a "mere" user, who may be ill-advised, than to a dealer making a profit from the weaknesses of others. Offenses treated under the vice model (partial prohibition) range from gambling--the person who takes illegal bets is guilty of a crime while the person who places them is not--to the offense of selling new automobiles not equipped with seat belts--the seller, not the buyer, is guilty of an offense. Even Prohibition in 1919 never criminalized the possession or use of alcohol, only its manufacture and sale.

EFFECTS OF PARTIAL PROHIBITION

Probably the most important fact about a policy of prohibition of supply only is that where it has been adopted it has apparently not led to appreciably higher levels of marijuana use than would have existed if use were also prohibited. The National Commission on Marijuana and Drug Abuse's speculations about the lack of change in use patterns resulting from repeal of prohibitions on use have been confirmed by data since 1972. Reports from California, Oregon, and Maine indicate no appreciable increase in use following decriminalization of use, at least in the short term.

Oregon, the first state to repeal prohibition of use (in October 1973) has been studied in a series of Drug Abuse Council surveys (National Governors' Conference, 1977). Surveys in 1974 and 1975 showed no major increase following decriminalization. While the percentage of adults who were current users had increased by January 1977 (from 20 to 24 percent), use had increased similarly nationwide in the same period, suggesting that the causes for the adult increase in Oregon were the same as those for increases in the rest of the country rather than the result of changes in the law. Indeed, the percentage of adult ever-users in Oregon in 1976 (24 percent) was lower than the average percentage of adult ever-users in the western United States (28 percent) in 1975-1976, although higher than the national average (21.3 percent). (It should be noted that aggregate use rates in the western United States are heavily weighted by use rates in California, the largest western state, which had relatively high rates even prior to the state repeal of prohibition of use.) That the increase in use in Oregon from 1973 to 1976 was probably not due to the new law is suggested by other survey data. Only a small proportion of non-users said fear of legal prosecution was a reason for nonuse in 1974, 1975, and 1976 (National Governors' Conference, 1977). On the question of the fear of health dangers, Drug Abuse Council survey data show that such fear decreased significantly over those years but has increased since 1976.

The state of Maine, which repealed criminal penalties for marijuana use in May 1976, surveyed the effects of legislation in July and August 1978 (State of Maine Department of Human Services, 1979). Its study concluded that the change from criminal to civil penalties has not caused a large increase in marijuana use: less than 1 percent of all adults and 3.1 percent of all high school students reported any increase in their use as a result of the new law; 3.5 percent of adult regular users and 7 percent of high school regular users reported any increase in their use directly attributable to the change in the law. There is also preliminary evidence, based on a nationwide study of high school students between 1975 and 1979, that "any increase in marijuana use in the decriminalized states, taken as a group, was equal to or less than the increases being observed in the rest of the country where decriminalization was not taking place" (Johnston, 1980:5). It could be argued that because de facto repeal of prohibition of use has been taking place throughout the country, one should not expect to see larger increases in use in states that legally decriminalize than in others. Even if this is true, however, the important point is that the legal change to decriminalization does not, in itself, appear to lead to increases in use.

This lack of change is not particularly surprising. The statistical chance that any person would be apprehended for his or her use is, in fact, extremely low throughout the United States (though, as we note below, the large number of users is sufficient to generate a substantial volume of arrests in states that do prohibit use). As a result, it is hard to imagine that the deterrent effect of prohibition laws on any given user would be very great.

It has been suggested that repeal of government prohibitions might change attitudes related to health or morals, perhaps symbolizing that health officials certify marijuana use to be safe. The absence of large increases in marijuana use in repeal states, however, indicates that either the change in policy has not had such a symbolic effect, or that, if it has, its causal significance is not appreciable--though it must be acknowledged that changes of this type might take generations to occur.

COSTS OF PROHIBITION OF USE

The costs of policies directed at the user are not negligible, although actual savings in law enforcement costs attributable to repeal of prohibition of use per se are difficult to estimate. The difficulty arises in part because marijuana arrests have decreased nationally in recent years, reflecting the overall tendency to relax enforcement of marijuana laws, and that change could lead to inaccurate estimates of the impact of repeal. Nevertheless, reduced law enforcement activities seem to have led to substantial savings in states that have repealed laws that prohibit use.

California made a careful study of the economic impact of its law repealing prohibition of use, which went into effect in January 1976 (State Office of Narcotics and Drug Abuse, 1977). The law reduced the penalty for personal possession of one ounce or less of marijuana from a possible felony to a citable misdemeanor, punishable as an infraction with a maximum fine of $100 without regard to prior possession offenses. Criminal custody, booking, and pretrial incarceration procedures were eliminated. Possession of more than one ounce was also made a misdemeanor, with a maximum fine of $500, six months in jail, or both. According to the study, these changes resulted in a 74 percent reduction in what the state had been spending yearly to enforce its marijuana laws. (Estimates of what the state had been spending ranged from $35 million to more than $100 million yearly; see National Governors' Conference, 1977.)

In addition to its economic benefits, repealing prohibition of use saves the social costs of criminalizing the marijuana user. In recent years, close to 400,000 people have been arrested each year for marijuana-related offenses despite the general nonenforcement of criminal sanctions for use (Federal Bureau of Investigation, 1980). Only a small fraction of the arrests are made under federal law, largely for importation of marijuana. About 85 percent of all marijuana-related arrests are for possession, usually of one ounce or less (see, e.g., State Office of Narcotics and Drug Abuse, 1977).

A study by the National Commission on Marijuana and Drug Abuse of a sample consisting of some 3,000 of the people arrested for marijuana-related offenses in 1970 indicated that the marijuana arrest was usually the arrestee's first experience with the criminal justice system, particularly among juveniles (National Commission on Marijuana and Drug Abuse, 1972). Yet, "it is standard practice for law enforcement agencies to report such offenses to prospective employers, licensing agencies, and other authorities as 'narcotic drug arrests' " (testimony of Jay Miller, American Civil Liberties Union, to the Select Committee on Narcotics Abuse and Control, 1977). Thus young users, who are often otherwise law-abiding people, are subject to an arrest record, or even a prison term, with implications extending into many aspects of their lives.

Alienation from the rule of law in democratic society may be the most serious cost of current marijuana laws. The National Commission on Marijuana and Drug Abuse was concerned that young people who see no rational basis for the legal distinction between alcohol and marijuana may become cynical about America's political institutions and democratic process. The American Bar Association report (printed in Select Committee on Narcotics and Drug Abuse, 1977) concurs in the view that marijuana laws that criminalize the millions of Americans who have used marijuana engender disrespect for the law.

PUBLIC ATTITUDES TOWARD PARTIAL PROHIBITION

Although the National Commission on Marijuana and Drug Abuse concluded that prohibition of supply only would be a better policy than prohibition of supply and use, it felt that a serious disadvantage of such a course would be the upset and moral outrage such a policy would engender. Hindsight now shows that the Commission was mistaken in predicting a strong uniform public reaction to the adoption of partial prohibition policies. Experience since 1973 has shown that repeal of criminal penalties for use of marijuana has not been accompanied by massive public protest in the states in which it occurred and, in fact, has had the approval of the majority of citizens in those states (National Governors' Conference, 1977).

Nationally, attitude trends are consistent with the experience of the repeal states. Roffman (1978) reports that public opinion surveys indicate a slowly increasing preference for a reduction in penalties for marijuana offenses; a 1975 national survey (National Institute on Drug Abuse, 1975-1976) found that 52 percent of American adults favored only a fine or probation for small marijuana offenses; and a 1977 Gallup poll showed that 28 percent of the public favored legalization, compared with 12 percent in 1969.

THE SUPPLY OF MARIJUANA: COMPARING PROHIBITED AND REGULATED MARKETS

Policy implementation does not occur in an ideal world. Prohibition of supply has not, in practice, meant that no one has had access to marijuana--though this may have been the intent of those who framed that law. Similarly, regulation of supply does not mean that everyone who uses marijuana will use it moderately, minimizing its harm. Prohibition of supply does make marijuana less accessible than it might otherwise be to a large number of Americans, and thus it almost certainly reduces the total amount of the drug used and the number of users. Such reduction is the purpose of a partial prohibition policy and to some extent it is accomplished. Arguments for a regulated, legal supply of marijuana are largely based on the social costs and incomplete effectiveness of prohibition of supply and on the belief that regulating rather than prohibiting the supply would not lead to an unacceptably large increase in use.

Under a regulatory policy, the cultivation, importation, manufacture, distribution, retailing, and, of course, use of marijuana would no longer be illegal per se. Within this broad category, specific policy options range from a virtual withdrawal of the government from marijuana control (allowing the drug to be freely produced, advertised, and sold, very much as coffee is today--but protecting the consumer against harmful adulterants), to a carefully controlled system of licensing, to a government monopoly on retail sales, wholesale distribution, or manufacture of marijuana. Thus, controls might be placed on such factors as quality, potency, amount purchased, time and place of sales, age of buyers, etc. If marijuana were regulated as is alcohol, restrictions would derive from federal, state, or local statutes, with the majority of them not at the federal level. Regulations might also include legally fixed prices--as in state-controlled alcohol beverage retailing or as a consequence of the levying of excise taxes.

The specific form and content of any proposed regulatory system are very important for those faced with the decision as to whether and under what conditions to remove penalties for the distribution of marijuana, but such details are beyond the scope of this report.

The advantages of a policy of regulation include the disappearance of most illegal market activity, the savings in economic and social costs of law enforcement directed against illegal supply systems, better controls over the quality and safety of the product, and, possibly, increased credibility for warnings about risks. The major disadvantages are a consequence of increased marijuana use--increases in harm to physical health and to individual development and behavior.

COSTS OF PROHIBITION OF SUPPLY

The number of arrests for violations related to supply is much lower than for those related to use. But enforcement of prohibition of supply is far more costly per arrest. Long undercover investigations, the purchase of expensive hardware, and the major consumption of trial and correctional resources are largely attributable to the prohibition of supply.

The National Institute on Drug Abuse (1975) estimated that in 1974 costs for enforcement of marijuana laws totaled $600 million for state and local agencies. If we extrapolate from the California data (State Office of Narcotics and Drug Abuse, 1977), about three-fourths of the total is spent enforcing the law against marijuana supply. The total federal drug abuse law enforcement budget was more than $400 million in 1979, about half of which was the budget for the Drug Enforcement Administration. At the federal level, authorities do not break down their expenditures on enforcement between marijuana and other drugs; virtually all of the federal resources that are allocated to marijuana are spent in attempting to enforce the laws against supply.

The task of attempting to make the prohibition of supply effective is, of course, formidable. In 1969 Operation Intercept demonstrated the practical difficulty of sealing off the Mexican border. In the weeks the operation lasted, hundreds of thousands of vehicles and passengers were searched every day; ensuing traffic jams caused expenditures by U.S. tourists and commuters to Mexico to drop 50-70 percent below normal (Kaplan, 1971). The situation was intolerable and the program was halted. However, the federal government has continued efforts to improve border surveillance and to penetrate trafficking networks. The White House Strategy Council on Drug Abuse (1979) notes that more than 5.6 million pounds of marijuana was seized at the Mexican border over a 12-month period in 1977-1978; a large increase over the 1.5 million pounds seized during the previous 12 months, "but a fraction of marijuana entering the country." Recently, the Council has suggested strengthening border surveillance by cooperative efforts of the Drug Enforcement Administration, the Customs Service, the Coast Guard, and the Department of State and by the use of the detection capabilities of the armed forces as well.

In our view, the prospects for major success in these ventures are not great. Nor is there much likelihood that some recently suggested measures against marijuana production outside the U.S. would make future prohibition of supply more effective. For example, the White House Strategy Council on Drug Abuse has supported crop eradication programs, provided that the proposed method of eradication is evaluated for possible health and environmental consequences and that a readily distinguishable marker is added to any chemical herbicides that are used, but the political obstacles to this course would be significant. Entirely apart from the views of producer nations, which are likely to be quite negative, the public is unlikely to support the use of chemicals of unknown toxicity on an import product, legal or not, that may be used by large numbers of Americans. And irrespective of the degree of success of controlling imports, the problem of domestic production under a policy of partial prohibition remains. Although the illegal domestic industry is thought to account for only about 15 percent of American marijuana consumption, marijuana grows easily in many parts of the United States. The National Commission on Marijuana and Drug Abuse cited a Department of Agriculture estimate that in 1972 there were 5 million acres containing wild marijuana in the United States and an undetermined but obviously growing number of acres under cultivation.

Law enforcement costs are by no means the only costs of prohibition of supply. There are large amounts of money being made in marijuana--which, like any illegal business, carries with it the likelihood of corruption of public officials and the loss of tax dollars. Violence is also a cost of attempting to prohibit marijuana supply; this problem is not confined to illegal marijuana production abroad. There has been violence in marijuana-growing regions in the United States. The extent of such violence is not known with any precision, but there have been popular press reports of kidnappings, assaults, burglaries, and homicides known to be connected with the marijuana business in northern California and elsewhere.

Another major cost of attempts to prohibit the supply of marijuana is related to the fact that many illegal sellers of marijuana also sell other illegal drugs, e.g., PCP, amphetamine, and barbiturates (Blum, 1971). It is likely, therefore, that prohibition of the supply of marijuana increases access to and use of other illegal drugs through the creation of an illegal marketing system for all drugs. Little is known about the structures and activities of illicit drug markets. It is clear,

TABLE 1 Lifetime Prevalence and Use in Past Month of Marijuana, 1971-1979, by Category of User (percentage)

Category of User	1971	1972	1974	1976	1977	1979
Youth: Ages 12-17						
Ever used	14.0	14.0	23.0	22.4	28.0	30.9
Used in past month	6.0	7.0	12.0	12.3	16.6	16.7
Young Adults: Ages 18-25						
Ever used	39.3	47.9	52.7	52.9	59.9	68.2
Used in past month	17.3	27.8	25.2	25.0	27.4	35.4
Older Adults: Ages 26+						
Ever used	9.2	7.4	9.9	12.9	15.3	19.6
Used in past month	1.3	2.5	2.0	3.5	3.3	6.0
(Number)	(3,186)	(3,265)	(4,022)	(3,576)	(4,594)	(7,224)

SOURCE: Fishburne et al. (1980).

however, that there are many small-scale marijuana dealers, that many sellers service only their friends and acquaintances, and that those who sell marijuana are thereby more likely to come into contact with users and sellers of more dangerous drugs, to use such drugs, and to make them available to their clientele (Blum, 1971). Moreover, there is reason to believe that marijuana sellers may become socialized into other illegal activities.

COSTS OF REGULATING SUPPLY

The wide availability and use of marijuana are not only major factors in the cost of attempts to prohibit the supply of the drug, they also have implications for the likely magnitude of increases in use that could be expected under a regulatory policy. Greater use of marijuana under a regulatory policy is regarded as the most significant cost of such a policy. In an analysis of this potential cost, however, it is important to note that under the present policy of prohibition, prevalence and frequency of marijuana use are substantial and have increased in recent years.*

A National Institute on Drug Abuse general household survey (Fishburne et al., 1980) shows that 35.4 percent of the 18-25-year-olds in the United States report having used marijuana in the month preceding the survey. Yearly surveys show a steady increase from 1971 to 1979 in the percentage of people who report having ever used marijuana as well as in the percentage of people who report being current users (see Table 1). These survey results (Fishburne et al., 1980) also indicate that between 1976 and 1977, the percentage of current users among 12-17-year-olds increased from 12.3 to 16.6 percent; this trend had leveled off by 1979 and has since shown a decline. In an annual survey of national samples of some 17,000 high school seniors, Johnston et al. (1982) found that 7.0 percent of the class of 1981 reported daily marijuana use, compared with 6.0 percent in 1975 and 10.7 percent in 1978, the peak year (see Table 2). There has been a similar trend in initial use at younger ages.

---

*The data indicating rates of use are based on self-reports; as such, their reliability and validity may be questioned. Nevertheless, as Radosevich et al. (1979) indicate, studies of questions on drug use have consistently demonstrated reliable responses within the same instrument and over time. Furthermore, there are indications that most drug surveys do not have serious validity problems (see Whitehead and Smart and Abelson and Atkinson, both cited in Radosevich et al., 1979; Johnston et al., 1982).

TABLE 2 Trends in Prevalence of Marijuana Use by High School Seniors (percentage)

Prevalence	Class 1975	1976	1977	1978	1979	1980	1981
Ever used	47.3	52.8	56.4	59.2	60.4	60.3	59.5
Used in last 12 months	40.0	44.5	47.6	50.2	50.8	48.8	46.1
Used in last 30 days	27.1	32.2	35.4	37.1	36.5	33.7	31.6
Used daily in last 30 days[a]	6.0	8.2	9.1	10.7	10.3	9.1	7.0

[a]Daily use defined as using marijuana on 20 or more occasions in the last 30 days.
SOURCE: Johnston et al. (1982).

Although the present policy of prohibition of supply is not preventing the current levels of marijuana use, including use among the very young, it is probable that most strategies under a regulatory policy would result in an overall increase in use. Even more important than overall use rates, however, are likely changes in consumption patterns; such patterns are the most difficult changes to predict. The smallest increases in numbers of users can be expected to occur among those to whom marijuana is now most readily available--the young. Johnston et al. (1982) found that close to 90 percent of the high school seniors in their national sample survey report that marijuana is "fairly easy" or "very easy" for them to get. This percentage remained relatively stable over the seven years, 1975-1981. At the same time, the reported availability of most other illegal drugs (except cocaine) declined considerably. For example, while 46.2 percent of the 1975 high school seniors said that LSD would be "fairly easy" or "very easy" to get, only 32.2 percent of the class of 1978 gave those responses. It would appear, therefore, that the reports of easy availability are not due to a tendency of adolescents to report any illegal drug as easy to get, but reflect their actual access to the drug. It might also be noted that only 13.9 percent of the class of 1978 reported having no friends who smoke marijuana; thus it is reasonable to expect that at least 86 percent have a factual basis for estimating the availability of the drug.

Other survey data corroborate these findings. Radosevich et al. (1979) report that a 1975 national survey by the Drug Abuse Council found that at least 70 percent of the high school students in their sample reported marijuana "easy to get," and O'Donnell et al. (1976) found similar results. There are no contrary reports for recent years. In sum, one can be reasonably confident that, at least with respect to older adolescents, the prohibition against supply does not succeed in suppressing access to marijuana. (The effect on price is discussed below.)

Regulation could be expected to provide the greatest increase in availability to those to whom the drug is now least available, i.e., older adults who are not in contact with marijuana sellers or a drug-using subculture and who are most likely to avoid illegal "connections."

It has been argued that a serious cost of the adoption of a regulatory policy for marijuana is the likelihood that such a change might delude many people into believing that the drug is safe. As noted above, there is no indication that the elimination of penalties for marijuana use has caused the drug to be regarded as any less dangerous. Moreover, alcohol and tobacco are almost universally regarded as involving risks to health, and these drugs are already made available under regulatory systems.

To the extent that marijuana use causes harm, one is necessarily concerned about policy changes that will lead to increases in use. As we have noted, however, it is a fact that marijuana is already widely available despite the legal prohibition of supply and that, despite the best efforts of government under any foreseeable set of conditions, it will continue to be. Though a regulatory policy would increase the availability of the drug, estimates of the size of these increases, and associated increases in harm, must be weighed against estimates of the costs and weaknesses of continuing prohibitions of supply. In pragmatic terms, the issue is whether more harm would be done, overall, by retaining the partly effective, costly prohibition of supply or by moving to a system of legalized regulated sales--wherein presumably more people would use more marijuana, but some of the costs imposed by prohibition of supply would be removed.

REGULATORY SYSTEMS: SOME CONCRETE ASPECTS

To this point, a policy of regulation has been discussed rather abstractly in contrast with the more concrete discussion of prohibition policies. Experimentation with varying systems of regulation followed by adjustment and readjustment based on experience would be necessary before those most appropriate for particular circumstances could be developed. This can be a complex matter. For instance, U.S. alcohol policy, developed with the repeal of Prohibition, consists of an umbrella of national policy and a wide variety of supporting state and local regulation. The national policy umbrella includes controls on importation, taxation, potency, packaging, labeling, advertising, use in federal jurisdictions (e.g., parks, military installations), and use in systems regulated by the federal government (e.g., air transportation); it also provides funds and guidelines for the treatment of casualties of excessive use. Under the umbrella policy, states and local jurisdictions regulate taxes, retail sales, hours of availability, age limits, and the like, where supply is legal, or prohibit sales entirely. Some states have monopoly systems for package sales, others use licensed private stores. Historically, under this system, the strictness of controls has reflected local sentiment about the consumption of alcohol. Although few "dry" jurisdictions exist today, various degrees of local "dryness" were quite widespread until very recently (National Research Council, 1981).

Controlling Use

A regulated system of marijuana sale might attempt to moderate use by inhibiting the frequency of use and the amounts used as well as by prescribing conditions of purchase and use. However, it is likely that under a regulatory system consumption would in great part be controlled by informal social norms--as it is today.

Manipulating the price of the drug is an obvious means of inhibiting use. It has been argued that most adults would be willing to pay a higher price for legal marijuana than they currently pay for illegal supplies in return for not having to seek out "connections" and being relieved of the feeling that they may be supporting organized crime. A high price would be comparatively more restrictive for young people--precisely those whom one would most want to discourage from use--since, though they seem affluent compared with young people in previous times, their budgets are in fact more constrained than those of adults. The possibility of illegal markets selling to young people remains, but today's kind of illegal market for marijuana would probably shrink greatly under a regulatory system in the same way that illegal alcohol distribution systems have become so scarce. Young users would be much more likely to gain access to marijuana by diversion from the legal market--as they do today for alcohol--or from homegrown plants than from a wholly illegal chain of distributors. Such a development would make marijuana selling a less profitable and status-producing occupation among the young.

It has been suggested that if legal limits were imposed on the potency of legally available marijuana, a substantial illegal market for high-potency forms of the drug, including hashish, would still exist. Since it is likely that there would continue to be some users who prefer high-potency forms of cannabis, this is a reasonable concern. But there is no compelling a priori reason to believe that a legal structure for retail marijuana sales, which includes limits on potency, would result in any increase in the availability and use of high-potency products.

Home Cultivation

Cultivation of marijuana by users is another issue that would have to be confronted in devising a regulatory system. Growing marijuana without payment of a tax might be treated as a revenue offense. Without criminal penalties or vigorous enforcement, however, deterrent effects would be minimal since marijuana can be grown indoors anywhere in the United States using artificial light--and at comparatively little expense. A recent British study of options for marijuana control (Logan, 1979) suggests that, from a law enforcement perspective, it is not feasible to attempt to control home cultivation. Whether users would take the trouble to grow their own marijuana would depend in part on the legal price. The relatively high prices that might be charged in order to discourage use and to increase revenues would also tend to encourage home cultivation. Whatever its disadvantages, however, the use of homegrown marijuana at least would not bring users into contact with those who illegally sell the drug. With respect to young people, moreover, marijuana under cultivation is much harder for children to hide from parents than is the purchased prepared drug, and cultivation by juveniles could remain illegal if age limits on use were imposed. Nonetheless, the treatment of home cultivation represents a major issue for the design of a regulatory system.

Public Education

Excessive use may be discouraged by policies aimed at public education and at the use of the media, including a ban on commercial advertising. Although information on how to use drugs, on drug hazards, and on the attributes of drugs is passed along most effectively through informal channels (see, e.g., Hanneman, 1972), media and education programs can make such information far more readily available.

Research on the communication of messages to the public has identified source credibility as a major factor contributing to the persuasive power of a message (McGuire, 1969). It appears that the public is now extremely wary of some government information programs that attempt to influence health behaviors. The credibility of the federal government may be especially suspect when it issues health warnings about an illegal substance that it is clearly trying to prohibit. Rosenthal (1979) asserts that distrust of the government and the medical establishment has grown because of past exaggerations and distortions of the effects of some mind-altering drugs.

Informal Social Controls

In an assessment of possibilities for governmental controls under a regulatory system, the operation of informal norms for controlling substance use practices must be taken into account (Maloff et al., 1980). National experience with alcohol use, for example, provides evidence that there are informal rituals and sanctions that generally encourage moderation in the use of recreational drugs. Moreover, moderation is encouraged when a drug is introduced gradually, that is, to a growing population of users, like marijuana in the 1960s and early 1970s. One might expect that when a new drug is introduced into a society, governmental control would be particularly important since no informal controls for teaching people appropriate rules for use would have developed. If a potent drug is made widely available precipitously and very cheaply to a novice population, severe societal disruptions may occur: for example, the gin epidemics of early eighteenth-century England (see Clark, 1976). Because in the past two decades informal norms for controlling marijuana use have spread in the United States under conditions of greatly increased availability of marijuana, there is reason to believe that widespread uncontrolled use would not occur under regulation. Indeed, regulation might facilitate patterns of controlled use by diminishing the "forbidden fruit" aspect of the drug and perhaps increasing the likelihood that an adolescent would be introduced to the drug through families and friends who practice moderate use, rather than through their heaviest-using, most drug-involved peers.

Relations Among States

As has historically been the case with respect to alcohol, state governments differ in their approaches to marijuana. So long as present federal law continues to prohibit cultivation and distribution of marijuana, states cannot adopt a regulatory system, although they are legally free to reduce or eliminate their own penalties for sale and are not compelled to enforce federal laws. If federal law were changed, however, the institution of a regulatory system in one state would have reverberations in other states. Residents of states that continued to prohibit marijuana could be expected to cross state lines to purchase the drug in a state with a regulated system, thus further compromising the ability of states to enforce prohibition of supply among its residents. Furthermore, states that attempted to curtail consumption by raising prices might find their populations turning to lower-cost marijuana from neighboring states with lower prices. This is a familiar situation. Large numbers of both cigarettes and guns are smuggled illegally into New York from other states. Moreover, New Yorkers may travel to New Jersey to gamble in a casino, or Virginians to the District of Columbia to buy cheaper liquor. It is difficult to see how state prohibitions could remain effective if the number of states with regulatory systems grew very large unless the changes occurred in only one region of the country. However, there may be advantages in permitting a state-by-state approach. Conditions governing the costs and benefits both of partial prohibition and of regulation vary among the states. In this area of uncertainty, we may learn from experiment. If one regulatory system proved successful, other states would be more likely to adopt similar systems; similarly, if it worked poorly in one state, other states would be less inclined to adopt a regulatory policy.

Effects on Foreign Relations

The 1961 Single Convention on Narcotic Drugs, which now obligates the U.S. government to prevent the importation of marijuana and to prohibit the adoption of a licensing system by any state, is a serious (although not an insurmountable) obstacle to the adoption of a federal regulatory policy and the development of state licensing. The treaty allows a signatory to terminate its adherence to the agreement at any time after two years from the date of the convention. Of course the general impact of any move to withdraw from the convention includes a broad foreign policy context, which is beyond the expertise of this Committee to judge.

CONCLUSIONS

For the last decade, concern with health hazards attributable to marijuana has been rising. The hearts, lungs, reproductive functions, and mental abilities of children have been reported to be threatened by marijuana, and such threats are not to be taken lightly. Heavy use by anyone or any use by growing children should be discouraged. Although conclusive evidence is lacking of major, long-term public health problems caused by marijuana, they are worrisome possibilities, and both the reports and the a priori likelihood of developmental damage to some young users makes marijuana use a cause for extreme concern.

At the same time, the effectiveness of the present federal policy of complete prohibition falls far short of its goal--preventing use. An estimated 55 million Americans have tried marijuana, federal enforcement of prohibition of use is virtually nonexistent, and 11 states have repealed criminal penalties for private possession of small amounts and for private use. It can no longer be argued that use would be much more widespread and the problematic effects greater today if the policy of complete prohibition did not exist: The existing evidence on policies of partial prohibition indicates that partial prohibition has been as effective in controlling consumption as complete prohibition and has entailed considerably smaller social, legal, and economic costs. On balance, therefore, we believe that a policy of partial prohibition is clearly preferable to a policy of complete prohibition of supply and use.

We believe, further, that current policies directed at controlling the supply of marijuana should be seriously reconsidered. The demonstrated ineffectiveness of control of use through prohibition of supply and the high costs of implementing such a policy make it very unlikely that any kind of partial prohibition policy will be effective in reducing marijuana use significantly below present levels. Moreover, it seems likely to us that removal of criminal sanctions will be given serious consideration by the federal government and by the states in the foreseeable future. Hence, a variety of alternative policies should be considered.

At this time, the form of specific alternatives to current policies and their probable effect on patterns of use cannot be determined with confidence. It is possible that, after careful study, all alternatives will turn out to have so many disadvantages that none could command public consensus. To maximize the likelihood of sound policy for the long run, however, further research should be conducted on the biological, behavioral, developmental, and social consequences of marijuana use, on the structure and operation of drug markets, and on the relations of various conditions of availability to patterns of use.

RECOMMENDATIONS FOR RESEARCH

HEALTH AND BEHAVIOR

The persistent concern about the health-related effects of marijuana requires both an immediate and a continuing response. First, as the report of the Institute of Medicine (1982:5) recommends, there should be "a greatly intensified and more comprehensive program of research into the effects of marijuana on the health of the American people." An important goal of this research program should be the identification of subgroups at high risk for physiological and psychological damage in relation to patterns of use and doses of marijuana. The report presents a detailed agenda of needed research. Second, to the extent that potential health hazards are identified, policy research should address possible safeguards and precautions to protect the user.

If marijuana use can be scientifically shown to entail grave risks--to the brain, the cardiovascular and respiratory systems, or to reproductive functions, for example--that are currently not known, it can be argued that, as was the case with cigarette smoking, knowledge of those effects will be more effective than criminal enforcement as a deterrent to use.

DRUG MARKETS

Research on the price elasticity of demand in legal and illegal markets is a clear priority. The result of such research will be important in determining the likelihood of controlling heavy use through price mechanisms and in computing the amount of money--if any--that could be realized in taxation of marijuana.

Present knowledge of the structure and activities of drug markets and networks is insufficient to allow prediction of the effects of policy changes on them. Research in this area is difficult but the questions are important. If many dealers who sell cocaine, PCP, amphetamines, and barbiturates as well as marijuana would be put out of business if marijuana were available through legal channels, it might result in a curtailed market for a variety of other drugs. On the other hand, it is also possible that the market structure is so loosely organized, and dealers so transiently involved, that removing marijuana from the illegal markets would have little effect. To be sure, much research on some of these questions could not be conducted unless a regulatory system were in place in some state. Nonetheless, some research, particularly ethnographic and economic studies, should be undertaken now to discover the importance of marijuana profits to drug-dealing networks; the transiency, size, and nature of such networks; etc. It is essential for research in this area to be supported by appropriate government agencies.

EFFECTS ON USE

Although many questions remain to be answered before the most informed choices can be made between prohibiting and regulating supply, there are many things that cannot be known unless some jurisdiction tries a regulatory policy. Although adoption of a regulatory policy is likely to result in increased use, little is known about changes in patterns of use that are likely to result. If federal laws prohibiting supply are changed to allow states to license marijuana sales, epidemiological research programs must be ready to monitor any changes in use and their consequences. To do so, research should be organized and operating well in advance of any such policy changes in order to determine rates of use before the change. Although the shift in the law from complete to partial prohibition in 11 states has apparently had little effect on consumption patterns there, we do not know the degree to which legally available marijuana would attract a larger market. The impact on use of educational campaigns, health warnings, and informal social controls under a regulatory system should be investigated.

In the absence of the opportunity for states to adopt regulatory policies, there can only be educated guesses about which age groups are likely to increase use or whether individuals who now use marijuana will use more, etc. Meanwhile, every bit of analysis to predict the answers to these questions, by surveying public attitudes, assessing past experiences with the spread of drug use in society (e.g., alcohol use following the repeal of Prohibition), and critically reviewing the experience of other societies in which marijuana is more readily available, will be valuable.

Marijuana regulation would permit systematic provision of comprehensive, clearly communicated health warnings on package inserts or covers, in public health education, by medical practitioners, and by public health interest groups as well as by the government. The extent to which such warnings would have more credibility for users than current health warnings, generated in an atmosphere of prohibition, is an important subject for research. Despite widespread pessimism about the failures of drug education campaigns, there are encouraging results in educational approaches based on the Stanford Heart Disease Prevention Program experience. With appropriate, research-based models and techniques, public health education may be an attractive means for limiting excessive use (see, e.g., Maccoby, 1979).

REFERENCES

Abel, E.L. (1980) <u>Marijuana: The First Twelve Thousand Years</u>. New York and London: Plenum Press.

Beachy, G.M., Petersen, D.M., and Pearson, F.S. (1979) Adolescent drug use and delinquency: a research note. <u>Journal of Psychedelic Drugs</u> 11(4):313-316.

Blum, R.H. (1971) Drug pushers: a collective portrait. <u>Trans-Action</u> 8:18-21.

<u>Congressional Digest</u> (1979) Summary of federal and state laws. 58(2):37-38.

Clark, N.H. (1976) <u>Deliver Us From Evil: An Interpretation of American Prohibition</u>. New York: Norton.

Federal Bureau of Investigation (1980) <u>Uniform Crime Reports for the United States: 1980</u>. Available from the Superintendent of Documents, U.S. Government Printing Office. Washington, D.C.: U.S. Department of Justice.

Fishburne, P., Abelson, H., and Cisin, I. (1980) <u>National Survey on Drug Abuse: Main Findings 1979</u>. National Institute on Drug Abuse, DHHS Publication No. (ADM) 80-976. Washington, D.C.: U.S. Government Printing Office.

Fried, P.A. (1977) Behavioral and electroencephalographic correlates of marijuana: a review. <u>Behavioral Biology</u> 21(2):163-196.

Hanneman, G.J. (1972) <u>Dissemination of Drug Related Information</u>. Communication Research Program. Storrs: University of Connecticut.

Hochman, J.S., and Brill, N.Q. (1973) Chronic marijuana use and psychosocial adaptation. <u>American Journal of Psychiatry</u> 130(2):132-140.

Institute of Medicine (1982) <u>Marijuana and Health</u>. Report of the Committee to Study the Health-Related Effects of Cannabis and Its Derivatives. Washington, D.C.: National Academy Press.

Johnston, L. (1980) Marijuana Use and the Effects of Marijuana Decriminalization. Testimony delivered at hearings on the effects of marijuana, Subcommittee on Criminal Justice, Senate Judiciary Committee, January 16, Washington, D.C.

Johnston, L.D., Bachman, J.G., and O'Malley, P.M. (1982) <u>Student Drug Use in America 1975-1981</u>. National Institute on Drug Abuse. Available from the Superintendent of Documents, U.S. Government Printing Office. Washington, D.C.: U.S. Department of Health and Human Services.

REFERENCES

Kaplan, J. (1971) *Marijuana--The New Prohibition*. New York: World Publishing Co.

Logan, F. (1979) *Cannabis: Options for Control*. London: Quartermaine House.

Maccoby, N. (1979) Promoting Positive Health-Related Behavior in Adults. Paper presented at Fourth Vermont Conference on Primary Prevention of Psychopathology.

Maloff, D.R., Becker, H.S., Fonaroff, A., and Rodin, J. (1980) Informal social controls and their influence on substance use. Pp. 5-35 in D.R. Maloff and P.K. Levison, eds., *Issues in Controlled Substance Use*. Committee on Substance Abuse and Habitual Behavior, National Research Council. Washington, D.C.: National Academy of Sciences.

McGuire, W.J. (1969) The nature of attitudes and attitude change. In G. Lindzey and E. Aronson, eds., *The Handbook of Social Psychology*, Vol. 3. Menlo Park, Calif.: Addison-Wesley Publishing Co.

Nahas, G. (1977) Biomedical aspects of cannabis usage. *United Nations Bulletin on Narcotics* 29 (2):13-27.

National Commission on Marijuana and Drug Abuse (1972) *Marijuana: A Signal of Misunderstanding*. Washington, D.C.: U.S. Government Printing Office. [Reprinted as a Signet Special. New York: New American Library]

National Commission on Marijuana and Drug Abuse (1973) *Drug Use in America: Problem in Perspective*. Washington, D.C.: U.S. Government Printing Office.

National Governors' Conference (1977) *Marijuana: A Study of State Policies and Penalties*. Washington, D.C.: Center for Policy Research and Analysis.

National Institute on Drug Abuse (1975) Training the human. *Resources Bulletin* 1(3).

National Institute on Drug Abuse (1975-1976) *Nonmedical Use of Psychoactive Substances*. Washington, D.C.: U.S. Department of Health, Education, and Welfare.

National Institute on Drug Abuse (1979) *Seventh Annual Report on Marijuana and Health*. Available from the Superintendent of Documents, U.S. Government Printing Office. Washington, D.C.: U.S. Department of Health, Education, and Welfare.

National Institute on Drug Abuse (1980) *Eighth Annual Report on Marijuana and Health*. Available from the Superintendent of Documents, U.S. Government Printing Office. Washington, D.C.: U.S. Department of Health, Education, and Welfare.

REFERENCES

National Organization for the Reform of Marijuana Laws and Center for the Study of Non-Medical Drug Use (1979) The Marijuana Laws; State and Federal Penalties. Washington, D.C.

National Research Council (1981) Alcohol and Public Policy: Beyond the Shadow of Prohibition. M.H. Moore and D.R. Gerstein, eds. Panel on Alternative Policies Affecting the Prevention of Alcohol Abuse and Alcoholism, Committee on Substance Abuse and Habitual Behavior, National Research Council. Washington, D.C.: National Academy Press.

O'Donnell, J.A., Voss, H.L., Clayton, R.R., Slatin, G.L., and Room, R.G.W. (1976) Young Men and Drugs--A Nationwide Survey. National Institute on Drug Abuse Monograph Series No. 5. Available from the Superintendent of Documents, U.S. Government Printing Office. Washington, D.C.: U.S. Department of Health, Education, and Welfare.

Radosevich, M., Lanza-Kaduce, L., Akers, R.L., and Krohn, M.D. (1979) The sociology of adolescent drug and drinking behavior: a review of the state of the field; part 1. Deviant Behavior 1:15-35.

Roffman, R. (1978) Marijuana and its control in the late 1970s. Contemporary Drug Problems 6 (4):533-552.

Rosenthal, M. (1979) Partial prohibition of nonmedical use of mind-altering drugs: proposal for change. Houston Law Review 16:603-665.

Select Committee on Narcotics Abuse and Control (1977) Hearings: Decriminalization of Marijuana. House of Representatives, 95th Congress, March 14-16, 1977. Washington, D.C.: U.S. Government Printing Office.

State of Maine Department of Human Services (1979) An Evaluation of the Decriminalization of Marijuana in Maine--1978. Office of Alcoholism and Drug Abuse Prevention, Augusta,.

State Office of Narcotics and Drug Abuse (1977) A First Report of the Impact of California's New Marijuana Law (SB95). Sacramento, Calif.

Tashkin, D., et al. (1978) Cannabis, 1977. Annals of Internal Medicine 89:539-549.

White House Strategy Council on Drug Abuse (1979) Federal Strategy for Drug Abuse and Drug Traffic Prevention, 1979. Washington, D.C.: U.S. Government Printing Office.

APPENDIX: SUMMARY OF MARIJUANA AND HEALTH

The Institute of Medicine (IOM) of the National Academy of Sciences has conducted a 15-month study of the health-related effects of marijuana, at the request of the Secretary of Health and Human Services and the Director of the National Institutes of Health. The IOM appointed a 22-member committee to:

- analyze existing scientific evidence bearing on the possible hazards to the health and safety of users of marijuana;
- analyze data concerning the possible therapeutic value and health benefits of marijuana;
- assess federal research programs in marijuana;
- identify promising new research directions, and make sugggestions to improve the quality and usefulness of future research; and
- draw conclusions from this review that would accurately assess the limits of present knowledge and thereby provide a factual, scientific basis for the development of future government policy.

This assessment of knowledge of the health-related effects of marijuana is important and timely because marijuana is now the most widely used of all the illicit drugs available in the United States. In 1979, more than 50 million persons had tried it at least once. There has been a steep rise in its use during the past decade, particularly among adolescents and young adults, although there has been a leveling-off in its overall use among high school seniors in the past 2 or 3 years and a small decline in the percentage of seniors who use it frequently. Although substantially more high school students have used alcohol than have ever used marijuana, more high school seniors use marijuana on a daily or near-daily basis (9 percent) than alcohol (6 percent). Much of the heavy use of marijuana, unlike alcohol, takes place in school, where effects on behavior, cognition, and psychomotor performance can be particularly disturbing. Unlike alcohol, which is rapidly metabolized and eliminated from the body, the psychoactive components of marijuana persist in the body for a long time. Similar to alcohol, continued use of marijuana may cause tolerance and dependence. For all these reasons, it is imperative that we have reliable and detailed information about the effects of marijuana use on health, both in the long and short term.

What, then, did we learn from our review of the published scientific literature? Numerous acute effects have been described in animals, in isolated cells and tissues, and in studies of human volunteers; clinical and epidemiological observations also have been reported. This information is briefly summarized in the following paragraphs.

EFFECTS ON THE NERVOUS SYSTEM AND ON BEHAVIOR

We can say with confidence that marijuana produces acute effects on the brain, including chemical and electrophysiological changes. Its most clearly established acute effects are on mental functions and behavior. With a severity directly related to dose, marijuana impairs motor coordination and affects tracking ability and sensory and perceptual functions important for safe driving and the operation of other machines; it also impairs short-term memory and slows learning. Other acute effects include feelings of euphoria and other mood changes, but there also are disturbing mental phenomena, such as brief periods of anxiety, confusion, or psychosis.

There is not yet any conclusive evidence as to whether prolonged use of marijuana causes permanent changes in the nervous system or sustained impairment of brain function and behavior in human beings. In a few unconfirmed studies in experimental animals, impairment of learning and changes in electrical brain-wave recordings have been observed several months after the cessation of chronic administration of marijuana. In the judgment of the committee, widely cited studies purporting to demonstrate that marijuana affects the gross and microscopic structure of the human or monkey brain are not convincing; much more work is needed to settle this important point.

Chronic relatively heavy use of marijuana is associated with behavioral dysfunction and mental disorders in human beings, but available evidence does not establish if marijuana use under these circumstances is a cause or a result of the mental condition. There are similar problems in interpreting the evidence linking the use of marijuana to subsequent use of other illicit drugs, such as heroin or cocaine. Association does not prove a causal relation, and the use of marijuana may merely be symptomatic of an underlying disposition to use psychoactive drugs rather than a "stepping stone" to involvement with more dangerous substances. It is also difficult to sort out the relationship between use of marijuana and the complex symptoms known as the amotivational syndrome. Self-selection and effects of the drug are probably both contributing to the motivational problems seen in some chronic users of marijuana.

Thus, the long-term effects of marijuana on the human brain and on human behavior remain to be defined. Although we have no convincing evidence thus far of any effects persisting in human beings after cessation of drug use, there may well be subtle but important physical and psychological consequences that have not been recognized.

EFFECTS ON THE CARDIOVASCULAR AND RESPIRATORY SYSTEMS

There is good evidence that the smoking of marijuana usually causes acute changes in the heart and circulation that are characteristic of stress, but there is no evidence to indicate that a permanently deleterious effect on the normal cardiovascular system occurs. There is good evidence to show that marijuana increases the work of the heart, usually by raising heart rate and, in some persons, by raising blood pressure. This rise in workload poses a threat to patients with hypertension, cerebrovascular disease, and coronary atherosclerosis.

Acute exposure to marijuana smoke generally elicits broncho-dilation; chronic heavy smoking of marijuana causes inflammation and pre-neoplastic changes in the airways, similar to those produced by smoking of tobacco. Marijuana smoke is a complex mixture that not only has many chemical components (including carbon monoxide and "tar") and biological effects similar to those of tobacco smoke, but also some unique ingredients. This suggests the strong possibility that prolonged heavy smoking of marijuana, like tobacco, will lead to cancer of the respiratory tract and to serious impairment of lung function. Although there is evidence of impaired lung function in chronic smokers, no direct confirmation of the likelihood of cancer has yet been provided, possibly because marijuana has been widely smoked in this country for only about 20 years, and data have not been collected systematically in other countries with a much longer history of heavy marijuana use.

EFFECTS ON THE REPRODUCTIVE SYSTEM AND ON CHROMOSOMES

Although studies in animals have shown that delta-9-THC (the major psychoactive constituent of marijuana) lowers the concentration in blood serum of pituitary hormones (gonadotropins) that control reproductive functions, it is not known if there is a direct effect on reproductive tissues. Delta-9-THC appears to have a modest reversible suppressive effect on sperm production in men, but there is no proof that it has a deleterious effect on male fertility. Effects on human female hormonal function have been reported, but the evidence is not convincing. However, there is convincing evidence that marijuana interferes with ovulation in female monkeys. No satisfactory studies of the relation between use of marijuana and female fertility and child-bearing have been carried out. Although delta-9-THC is known to cross the placenta readily and to cause birth defects when administered in large doses to experimental animals, no adequate clinical studies have been carried out to determine if marijuana use can harm the human fetus. There is no conclusive evidence of teratogenicity in human offspring, but a slowly developing or low-level effect might be undetected by the studies done so far. The effects of marijuana on reproductive function and on the fetus are unclear; they may prove to be negligible, but further research to establish or rule out such effects would be of great importance.

Extracts from marijuana smoke particulates ("tar") have been found to produce dose-related mutations in bacteria; however, delta-9-THC, by itself, is not mutagenic. Marijuana and delta-9-THC do not appear to break chromosomes, but marijuana may affect chromosome segregation during cell division, resulting in an abnormal number of chromosomes in daughter cells. Although these results are of concern, their clinical significance is unknown.

THE IMMUNE SYSTEM

Similar limitations exist in our understanding of the effects of marijuana on other body systems. For example, some studies of the immune system demonstrate a mild, immunosuppressant effect on human beings, but other studies show no effect.

THERAPEUTIC POTENTIAL

The committee also has examined the evidence on the therapeutic effects of marijuana in a variety of medical disorders. Preliminary studies suggest that marijuana and its derivatives or analogues might be useful in the treatment of the raised intraocular pressure of glaucoma, in the control of the severe nausea and vomiting caused by cancer chemotherapy, and in the treatment of asthma. There also is some preliminary evidence that a marijuana constituent (cannabidiol) might be helpful in the treatment of certain types of epileptic seizures, as well as for spastic disorders and other nervous system diseases. But, in these and all other conditions, much more work is needed. Because marijuana and delta-9-THC often produce troublesome psychotropic or cardiovascular side-effects that limit their therapeutic usefulness, particularly in older patients, the greatest therapeutic potential probably lies in the use of synthetic analogues of marijuana derivatives with higher ratios of therapeutic to undesirable effects.

THE NEED FOR MORE RESEARCH ON MARIJUANA

The explanation for all of these unanswered questions is insufficient research. We need to know much more about the matabolism of the various marijuana chemical compounds and their biologic effects. This will require many more studies in animals, with particular emphasis on subhuman primates. Basic pharmacologic information obtained in animal experiments will ultimately have to be tested in clinical studies on human beings.

Until 10 or 15 years ago, there was virtually no systematic, rigorously controlled research on the human health-related effects of marijuana and its major constituents. Even now, when standardized marijuana and pure synthetic cannabinoids are available for experimental studies, and good qualitative methods exist for the measurement of delta-9-THC and its metabolites in body fluids, well-designed studies on human beings are relatively few. There are difficulties in studying the clinical effects of marijuana in human beings, particularly the effects of long-term use. And yet, without such studies the debate about the safety or hazard of marijuana will remain unresolved. Prospective cohort studies, as well as retrospective case-control studies, would be useful in identifying long-term behavioral and biological consequences of marijuana use.

The federal investment in research on the health-related effects of marijuana has been small, both in relation to the expenditure on other illicit drugs and in absolute terms. The committee considers the research particularly inadequate when viewed in light of the extent of marijuana use in this country, especially by young people. We believe there should be a greater investment in research on marijuana, and that investigator-initiated research grants should be the primary vehicle of support.

The committee considers all of the areas of research on marijuana that are supported by the National Institute on Drug Abuse to be important, but we did not judge the appropriateness of the allocation of resources among those areas, other than to conclude that there should be increased emphasis on studies in human beings and other primates. Recommendations for future research are presented at the end of Chapters 1-7 of this report.

CONCLUSIONS

The scientific evidence published to date indicates that marijuana has a broad range of psychological and biological effects, some of which, at least under certain conditions, are harmful to human health. Unfortunately, the available information does not tell us how serious this risk may be.

The major conclusion is that what little we know for certain about the effects of marijuana on human health--and all that we have reason to suspect--justifies serious national concern. Of no less concern is the extent of our ignorance about many of the most basic and important questions about the drug. Our major recommendation is that there be a greatly intensified and more comprehensive program of research into the effects of marijuana on the health of the American people.